CW00701150

Emergency First Aid a
including AED

Emergency First Aid at Work is published by: **Nuco Training Ltd**

UNIT TITLE: EMERGENCY FIRST AID IN THE WORKPLACE

LEARNING OUTCOMES	ASSESSMENT CRITERIA
1. Understand the role and responsibilities of a first aider	**1.1** Identify the role and responsibilities of a first aider
	1.2 Identify how to minimise the risk of infection to self and others
	1.3 Identify the need for consent to provide first aid
2. Be able to assess an emergency situation safely	**2.1** Conduct a scene survey
	2.2 Conduct a primary survey of a casualty
	2.3 Summon appropriate assistance when necessary
3. Be able to provide first aid to an unresponsive casualty	**3.1** Identify when to administer cardiopulmonary resuscitation (CPR)
	3.2 Demonstrate adult CPR using a manikin
	3.3 Identify when to place a casualty into the recovery position
	3.4 Demonstrate how to place a casualty into the recovery position
	3.5 Demonstrate continual monitoring of breathing whilst the casualty is in the recovery position
	3.6 Identify how to administer first aid to a casualty who is experiencing a seizure
4. Be able to provide first aid to a casualty who is choking	**4.1** Identify when a casualty is choking
	4.2 Demonstrate how to administer first aid to a casualty who is choking
5. Be able to provide first aid to a casualty with external bleeding	**5.1** Identify whether external bleeding is life-threatening
	5.2 Demonstrate how to administer first aid to a casualty with external bleeding
6. Know how to provide first aid to a casualty who is suffering from shock	**6.1** Recognise when a casualty is suffering from shock
	6.2 Identify how to administer first aid to a casualty who is suffering from shock
7. Know how to provide first aid to a casualty with minor injuries	**7.1** Identify how to administer first aid to a casualty with: • Small cuts • Grazes • Bruises • Small splinters • Nosebleeds
	7.2 Identify how to administer first aid to a casualty with minor burns and scalds

In all of our lives, whether at work, home or at play, it is essential that we all know how to assist someone who is sick, or has been injured.

First aid, as the term implies, is the initial treatment given to someone who is injured or sick, prior to professional medical assistance arriving and taking over from you.

By reading this manual, it will not make you a doctor, paramedic or nurse, but by applying common sense and some basic life support skills, as well as providing care and confidence in your treatment for the casualty, you will learn skills that will enhance their well-being and in some very serious cases, possibly save their life.

Your prompt, safe and effective treatment could make a difference between life and death.

As a First Aider, your priorities for the casualty fall into the following categories:

PRESERVE life

ALLEVIATE suffering

PREVENT further illness or injury

PROMOTE recovery

For instance, if your casualty is suffering major blood loss as a result of a serious cut, then you can **preserve life** by offering treatment immediately and not waiting for professional help to sort it out for you. If you do nothing, then your casualty could bleed to death.

We can **alleviate suffering** by making the casualty more comfortable, reducing their pain levels and offering lots of care and attention.

We can **prevent further illness or injury** by applying a secure sterile dressing on the injured part in order to control the blood loss and prevent the risk of infection.

We can **promote recovery** by treating the casualty for shock and ringing for an ambulance.

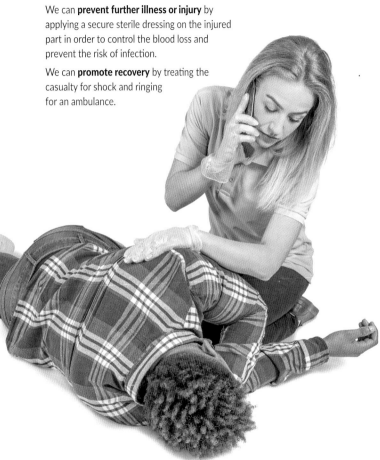

For some, you may have a responsibility in the workplace for first aid.

Should this be the case then you must be aware of legislation that ensures employers provide a duty of care, along with a first aid provision for their employees, as well as non-employees and contractors visiting their premises.

THE HEALTH AND SAFETY AT WORK ACT 1974

This Act, also abbreviated to **HSWA**, **HASWA** or **HASAWA**, is an Act of the Parliament of the United Kingdom that currently defines the fundamental structure and authority for the encouragement, regulation and enforcement of workplace health, safety and welfare within the United Kingdom.

The Act defines general duties on employers, employees, contractors, suppliers of goods and substances for use at work, persons in control of work premises, and those who manage and maintain them, and persons in general.

THE MANAGEMENT OF THE HEALTH AND SAFETY AT WORK REGULATIONS 1999

These Regulations generally make more explicit what employers are required to do to manage health and safety under the Health and Safety at Work Act. Like the Act, they apply to every work activity, including the provision of first aid.

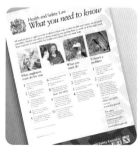

The main requirement for employers is to carry out a risk assessment. Employers with five or more employees need to record the significant findings of the risk assessment.

Risk assessment should be straightforward in a simple workplace such as a typical office. The HSE has guidance on these Regulations referred to as - Managing for Health and Safety (HSG65).

THE HEALTH AND SAFETY (FIRST AID) REGULATIONS 1981
(1982 IN NORTHERN IRELAND)

The Health and Safety (First-Aid) Regulations 1981 require employers to provide adequate and appropriate equipment, facilities and personnel to ensure their employees receive immediate attention if they are injured or taken ill at work.

FIRST AID AT WORK PROVISION

You should liaise with management and other First Aiders to ensure:

- There is an adequate number of First Aiders and Emergency First Aiders in place
- Appropriate equipment, kits and facilities are available
- A system is in place for incident and accident reporting

It is vital that a risk assessment of first aid needs is conducted to ensure that the correct level of provision is made.

Where the risk assessment identifies the need for people to be available for rendering first aid, then the employer should ensure that they are provided in sufficient numbers and at appropriate locations to enable first aid to be administered without delay, should the occasion arise.

Guidance on the Regulations for employers was introduced in October 2013 (L74 – Third edition).

The following table will guide you in ensuring that you have sufficient numbers of trained first aid personnel at your place of work.

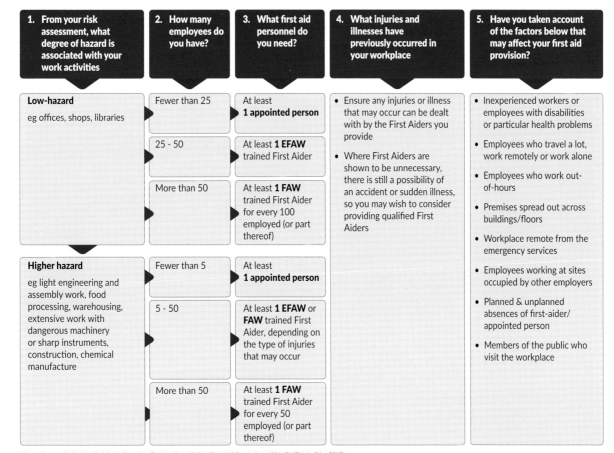

1. From your risk assessment, what degree of hazard is associated with your work activities	2. How many employees do you have?	3. What first aid personnel do you need?	4. What injuries and illnesses have previously occurred in your workplace	5. Have you taken account of the factors below that may affect your first aid provision?
Low-hazard eg offices, shops, libraries	Fewer than 25	At least **1 appointed person**	• Ensure any injuries or illness that may occur can be dealt with by the First Aiders you provide • Where First Aiders are shown to be unnecessary, there is still a possibility of an accident or sudden illness, so you may wish to consider providing qualified First Aiders	• Inexperienced workers or employees with disabilities or particular health problems • Employees who travel a lot, work remotely or work alone • Employees who work out-of-hours • Premises spread out across buildings/floors • Workplace remote from the emergency services • Employees working at sites occupied by other employers • Planned & unplanned absences of first-aider/ appointed person • Members of the public who visit the workplace
	25 - 50	At least **1 EFAW** trained First Aider		
	More than 50	At least **1 FAW** trained First Aider for every 100 employed (or part thereof)		
Higher hazard eg light engineering and assembly work, food processing, warehousing, extensive work with dangerous machinery or sharp instruments, construction, chemical manufacture	Fewer than 5	At least **1 appointed person**		
	5 - 50	At least **1 EFAW** or **FAW** trained First Aider, depending on the type of injuries that may occur		
	More than 50	At least **1 FAW** trained First Aider for every 50 employed (or part thereof)		

Information supplied by Health & Safety Executive. The Health and Safety (First-Aid) Regulations 1981 L74 (Third edition 2013)

FIRST AID CONTAINERS

The minimum level of first aid equipment is a suitably stocked and properly identified first aid container.

Every employer should provide, for each work site, at least one first aid container supplied with a sufficient quantity of first aid materials suitable for the particular circumstances.

There is no mandatory list of items to be included in a first aid container. The decision on what to provide, will be influenced by the findings of the first aid needs assessment. As a guide, where work activities involve low hazards, a minimum stock of first aid items might be:

- **A leaflet giving general guidance on first aid**
- **20 individually wrapped sterile plasters** (assorted sizes) **appropriate to the type of work** (hypoallergenic plasters can be provided if necessary)
- **Two sterile eye pads**
- **Four individually wrapped triangular bandages, preferably sterile**
- **Six safety pins**
- **Two large sterile individually wrapped unmedicated wound dressings**
- **Six medium-sized individually wrapped un-medicated wound dressings**
- **A pair of disposable gloves**

This is a suggested contents list only.

The contents of first aid containers should be examined frequently and restocked soon after use.

PERSONAL PROTECTIVE EQUIPMENT (PPE)

Employers should supply adequate PPE stored near to the first aid supplies. Such equipment could include hand sanitiser, face masks, safety glasses, ear protection, hi-vis vests and flashlights. Employers should also advise First Aiders on what PPE should be worn in which circumstances, ensuring that the First Aider's safety is the priority.

ADDITIONAL FIRST AID MATERIALS AND EQUIPMENT

The needs assessment may indicate that additional materials and equipment are required, for example scissors, burns dressings, adhesive tape, disposable aprons and individually wrapped moist wipes. They may be kept in the first aid container if there is room, or stored separately.

If mains tap water is not readily available for eye irrigation, at least a litre of sterile water or sterile normal saline (0.9%) in sealed, disposable containers should be provided. Once the seal has been broken, containers should not be kept for re-use. Containers should not be used beyond their expiry date.

First Aid at Work does not include giving tablets or medicines to treat illness.

> It is recommended that tablets and medicines should not be kept in the first aid container.

The view of the Health and Safety Executive (HSE), is that the administration of medication by a First Aider is not part of a First Aid at Work training course, but you can assist an individual in taking it, if it is their own medication.

However, the one exception is heart attacks. Therefore, for heart attack management, the First Aider must be able to assist a casualty in taking one aspirin tablet (300mg) and ask them to chew it slowly, providing you are confident that the casualty is not allergic to it. If you are in any doubt, then you **MUST NOT** administer it. Aspirin **MUST NOT** be administered to anyone under the age of 16.

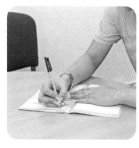

ACCIDENT AND INCIDENT REPORTING

Irrespective of the severity of the accident or incident, it is vital that all such occurrences be reported and filed by the employer.

Anyone can complete the accident book, and this book must comply with Data Protection legislation.

The accident book should be used as a useful reference for the purpose of ensuring that, where reasonably practicable, the same incident can be prevented from happening again.

An accident book can be purchased at most good book shops, or online from many first aid supply shops.

The information that should be recorded includes:

- **The date, time and place of the incident**
- **Name and job of the injured or ill person**
- **Details of the injury/illness and what first aid was given**
- **What happened to the casualty immediately afterwards?** (e.g. went back to work, went home, went to hospital)
- **Name and signature of the person reporting the incident**
- **The information must be kept in accordance with the Data Protection Act 2018**

Where the incident is of a severe nature, then the employer must comply with RIDDOR 2013.

> **Online electronic reporting is an acceptable form of recording accidents and incidents.**

RIDDOR is the law that requires employers, and other people in control of work premises, to report and keep records of:

- **Work-related accidents which cause death**
- **Work-related accidents which cause certain serious injuries** (reportable injuries)
- **Diagnosed cases of certain industrial diseases**
- **Certain 'dangerous occurrences'** (incidents with the potential to cause harm)

There are also special requirements for gas incidents.

Reporting certain incidents is a legal requirement. The report informs the enforcing authorities (HSE, local authorities and the Office for Rail Regulation (ORR)) about deaths, injuries, occupational diseases and dangerous occurrences, so they can identify where and how risks arise, and whether they need to be investigated.

Please visit www.hse.gov.uk/riddor/ for full details of what is reportable.

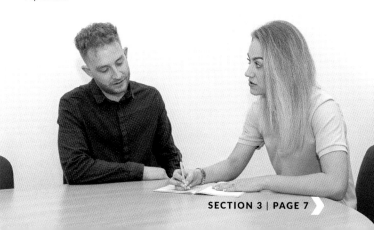

A First Aider has a number of responsibilities when dealing with an incident.

It is paramount that the incident is dealt with confidently and safely. The safety for all is important, including you, the casualty and any bystanders.

You must manage the incident and take control of the situation until professional medical help arrives and takes over. A bystander can be a great benefit to you, particularly if they are qualified in first aid, so don't be afraid to summon help.

A bystander can make a telephone call, get a first aid kit, return with the defibrillator if you have one, manage the crowd and traffic, and generally support you.

Your responsibilities can be broken up into the following categories:

- Arrival at the scene
- Dealing with casualties
- Casualty communication
- Contacting the emergency services
- Prioritise the first aid treatment
- Clearing up process and infection control

ARRIVAL AT THE SCENE

Make the area safe and gather as much information about the incident as you can.

The history of the incident and any casualty information about their illness or injury could help you decide your course of initial treatment.

CONSENT

A responsive adult must agree to receive first aid treatment. 'Expressed consent' means that the casualty gives their permission to receive care and treatment. To obtain consent, first identify yourself, tell them about your level of training and qualification and ask if it's ok to help them.

Implied consent means that permission to perform first aid care on an unresponsive casualty is assumed. This is based on the idea that a reasonable person would give their permission to receive lifesaving treatment if they were able to.

When caring for vulnerable groups such as children and the elderly then consent must be gained from a parent, family member or legal guardian. When life-threatening situations exist and the parent, family member or legal guardian is not available, you must provide first aid care based on implied consent.

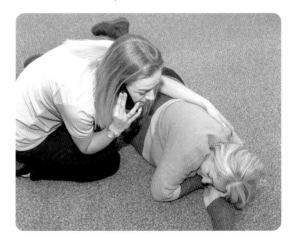

Common sense

It is necessary to apply common sense. Never attempt skills that exceed your training. Always ask a responsive casualty for permission before giving care.
Call for an ambulance immediately if no first aid treatment is given. Once you have started first aid, do not stop until medical help arrives and takes over from you.

Ensure you have help at hand.

You are almost certain to be feeling nervous and anxious yourself, but be as confident as you can, and take control of the situation.

DEALING WITH CASUALTIES

- Prioritise your treatment, particularly if you have multiple casualties
- Ensure safety for all
- Protect against contamination
- Be calm and confident
- Ensure that the appropriate emergency services have been called for

CASUALTY COMMUNICATION

Irrespective of the severity of the incident, your casualty could be in a state of shock and confusion. Therefore, your communication skills are critical in gaining their trust.

The groups that are most likely to be affected are children, the elderly, hearing impaired, visually impaired and non-English speaking casualties.

- Be honest about their condition, without exaggerating it
- Be careful of what you say which could distress them further
- Maintain eye contact when talking to them, and be aware of your body language. Their body language could tell you a lot about their condition
- Take your time when talking to them, particularly for the vulnerable groups such as the elderly and children
- Allow your casualty to explain how they are feeling. It could help you make a diagnosis enabling you to offer the right treatment
- In respect of their injury, avoid medical terms that they may not understand

L I O N E L

CONTACTING THE EMERGENCY SERVICES

As soon as you have identified the extent of the injury, then it may be necessary to contact the emergency services.
They can be contacted by dialling 999 or 112.

They will require vital information about the condition of the casualty so that the call can be prioritised.

Activate the speaker function on the phone to aid communication with the ambulance service.

They will also require specific details about the location of the incident. It is imperative that you have the full details of where you are, particularly if the premises are large and have multi-floors or other buildings to consider. Your bystander could manage this for you by meeting the emergency services and guiding them to the incident.

> **Only dial 999 if it is necessary and consider other services such as Police and Fire, dependent on the incident.**

Remember **LIONEL** when making this call:

L Location

I Incident

O Other services

N Number of casualties

E Extent of injuries

L Location - repeat

PRIORITISE YOUR FIRST AID TREATMENT

- **Breathing** – deal with casualties who are not breathing normally first
- **Bleeding** – deal with any major bleeding and treat the casualty for shock
- **Burns/breaks** – treat burns and immobilise any bone injuries
- **Other conditions** – treat appropriately

There are many conditions that could be deemed as life-threatening which require medication, such as diabetes, asthma and anaphylaxis. Where possible, you can assist your casualty by offering them their own medication if they have it with them.

Remember your priorities. Ensure that their airway remains open and that they are breathing normally for themselves.

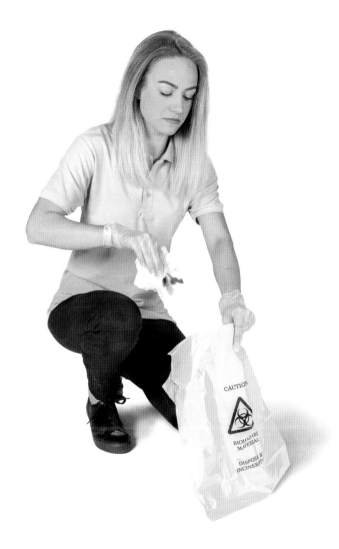

THE CLEARING UP PROCESS AND INFECTION CONTROL

You must minimise the risk of infection from the outset when dealing with any incident. This applies to you, the casualty, and any bystanders. Similarly, when the casualty has been treated it is vital that all soiled dressings etc, are disposed of correctly.

- Wash your hands and wear disposable gloves
- Avoid coughing and sneezing over the wound, and avoid touching it
- Dispose of all soiled dressings, including gloves, in an appropriately marked (orange/yellow) plastic bag
- Dispose of sharp items, including syringes and needles, in a purpose made sharps bin and dispose of it appropriately. It may mean taking it to your local hospital for correct disposal

Rescuers should take appropriate safety precautions where feasible, especially if the casualty is known to have a serious infection such as tuberculosis (TB), severe acute respiratory distress syndrome (SARS) or coronavirus (COVID-19).

During any outbreak of a highly infectious condition, protective precautions for the rescuer are essential.

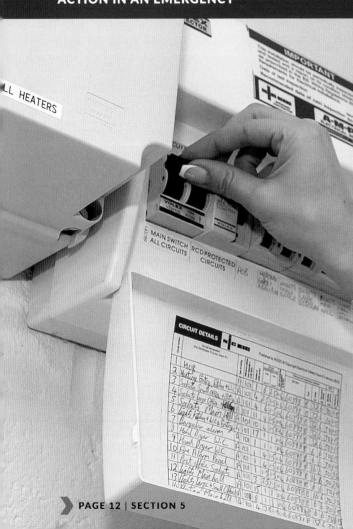

When confronted with any emergency situation, you need to take **SHAPE**!

S SAFETY AND PROTECTION

You must ensure the safety for all. Ensure you are adequately protected against the risk of infection and any other adverse element such as chemicals and gases

H HAZARDS

Be aware of potential hazards such as traffic, chemicals, fire, gas, electricity etc

A ASSESS THE SITUATION

Before rushing in to deal with an incident, you must assess the situation that you are confronted with

P PRIORITISE

Ensure you prioritise the injuries, particularly if you have multiple casualties

E ENVIRONMENT

Pay attention to the environment around you, and do not take risks. Jumping into water to save a drowning victim is not a good idea if you can't swim!

Irrespective of the incident you are confronted with, you must carry out an initial assessment of the situation including your casualty.

This is popularly known as the primary survey.
The contents of this survey can be remembered easily by using the mnemonic **DR ABC**.

DANGERS

The area must be safe before you offer your casualty any treatment. Safe for you primarily, not forgetting any bystanders and of course your casualty.

Failing to do this could result in you having more casualties to deal with, which could include yourself!

RESPONSE

Approach the casualty, ideally from their feet. This reduces the risk of the casualty hyper-extending their neck should they be responsive.

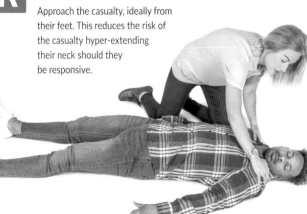

YOU CAN PERFORM A RESPONSIVE CHECK BY USING THE AVPU SCALE.

Alert If they are fully responsive, then ascertain the extent of their injury and deal with it appropriately.

Voice - "Are you all right?"
If they are not alert, then see if they will respond to a voice command.

Place your hands on their shoulders and gently shake them.
If they don't respond to a voice command, then try shaking them gently by the shoulders. NB: do not shake them if you suspect a spinal or head injury.

Unresponsive
If there is no response at all, they must be deemed as being unresponsive.

If your casualty responds, leave them in the position in which you find them providing there is no further danger. Try to find out what is wrong with them and treat accordingly.

Call for professional medical help if it is needed and reassess them regularly.

If you are on your own, you should shout for help. Ideally you should never leave your casualty on their own.

A bystander can be a great benefit to you such as:

- Calling for an ambulance
- Managing crowds and hazards
- Fetching the first aid kit and defibrillator if you have one
- Consoling relatives and friends
- Helping you if they are trained to do so
- Cleaning up
- A support for you

A AIRWAY

Turn the casualty onto their back and then open the airway using the head tilt and chin lift method:

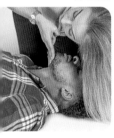

- **Place your hand on their forehead and gently tilt their head back**
- **With two fingertips under the point of their chin, lift the chin to open the airway**
- **Be careful not to press on the fleshy part under the chin as it could restrict the airway**

Support their head in this position in order to perform a breathing check.

B BREATHING

Look, listen and feel for normal breathing for no more than 10 seconds.

Look for chest movement

Listen at their mouth for breath sounds

Feel for air on your cheek

In the first few minutes after cardiac arrest, a casualty may be barely breathing, or taking infrequent, noisy, gasps. This is often termed agonal breathing or gasping, and must not be confused with normal breathing.

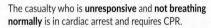

The casualty who is **unresponsive** and **not breathing normally** is in cardiac arrest and requires CPR.

Immediately following cardiac arrest blood flow to the brain is reduced to virtually zero, which may cause seizure-like episodes that may be confused with epilepsy.

You should be suspicious of cardiac arrest with any casualty that presents seizure like symptoms and carefully assess whether they are breathing normally.

C

If you have any doubt whether breathing is normal, act as if it is **not** normal and prepare to commence CPR.

CPR FOR A NON-BREATHING CASUALTY

If your casualty **is not breathing normally**, then an ambulance must be summoned immediately. Lone rescuers should utilise the speaker function on their phone when making this call. If you have a bystander at hand, ask them to make this important call so that you can commence cardiopulmonary resuscitation (CPR) without delay. (see page 21).

You can also ask your bystander to find and bring an Automated External Defibrillator (AED) to you, if one is available.

If your casualty is **breathing normally** and has no major physical trauma, they should be placed in the recovery position (see page 16) and an ambulance should be summoned.

If your casualty has sustained physical trauma, then the injuries should be treated accordingly and the casualty left in the position found. However, if you believe their airway is at risk, then the recovery position should be used.

Ensure that you monitor their breathing whilst in the recovery position.

If you are unsure about the extent of the injury, then you should perform a top-to-toe survey before placing them in the recovery position.

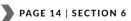

CASUALTY ASSESSMENT

As soon as you have completed your primary survey, and you have established that your casualty is breathing normally, you must then move on to the secondary assessment in order to determine the extent of their injury or illness, irrespective of whether they are responsive or not.

In order to make a diagnosis of their condition, there are three key factors to consider:

HISTORY

- Ask your casualty or bystanders what happened
- Examine the environment for obvious signs relating to the incident
- Ask your casualty about their condition. Do they have their own medication? Has it happened before? Where does it hurt? How painful is it?
- Ask the casualty their name. Is there any family present that could answer the questions about their condition?

SIGNS

- What can you see in respect of the injury or condition?
- Use all your other senses. What can you smell, hear and feel?

SYMPTOMS

This is how the casualty will be feeling, ask them how they are feeling.

- Communication is very important to ascertain the extent of their injury/illness

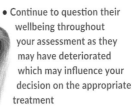

- Continue to question their wellbeing throughout your assessment as they may have deteriorated which may influence your decision on the appropriate treatment

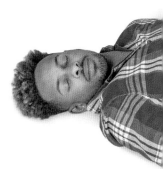

The recovery position

If your casualty is unresponsive, but breathing normally, with no evidence of major physical trauma, then your priority is to ensure that their airway is not compromised in any way and that it remains open.

Rather than leaving them on their back, or in a slumped position, then an effective way of achieving this is to place them in the recovery position.

Whilst the casualty remains in this position, it will allow vomit to drain from the mouth and prevent them from rolling onto their back should you have to leave them.

1 Remove the casualty's glasses, if present

2 Kneel beside the casualty and make sure that both their legs are straight

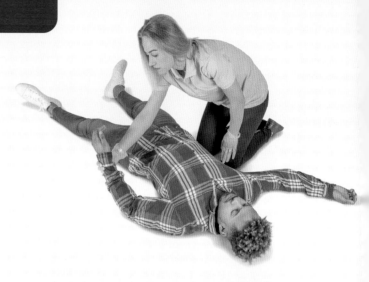

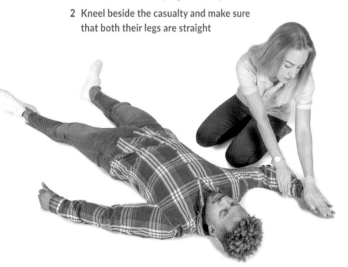

3 Place the arm nearest to you out at a right angle to their body, elbow bent with the hand palm-up. Do not force the arm, let it fall naturally, but close to this position

SUSPECTED SPINAL INJURY

If you suspect a spinal injury and you cannot maintain an open airway in the position you found them, care must be taken in moving them.

Keep the casualty's back straight and support the head throughout.

It would be extremely useful to have help in moving the casualty.

The trained person should assume control when moving them.

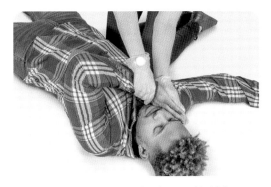

4 Bring the far arm across the chest, and hold the
   back of the hand against their cheek nearest to you

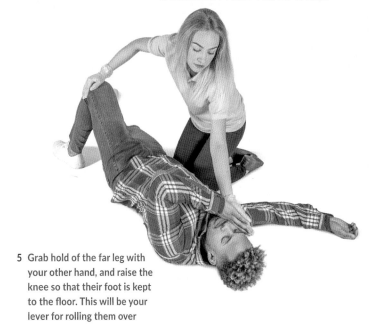

5 Grab hold of the far leg with
   your other hand, and raise the
   knee so that their foot is kept
   to the floor. This will be your
   lever for rolling them over

6 Keeping their hand pressed against their
   cheek, pull on the far leg to roll them
   towards you onto their side with their
   head supported all the way

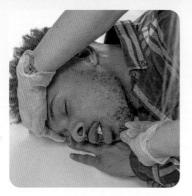

7 Tilt the head back to make sure that the airway remains open

8 If necessary, adjust the hand under their cheek to keep the head tilted and facing downwards to allow liquid material to drain from the mouth

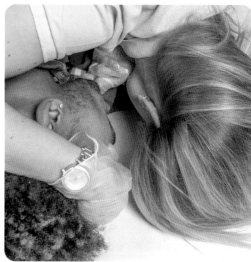

9 Adjust the upper leg so that both the hip and knee are bent at right angles

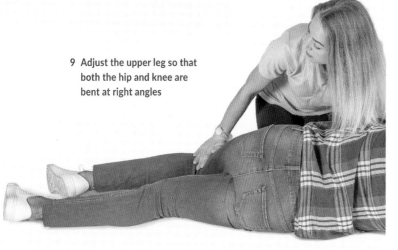

10 Check breathing regularly

SUSPECTED SPINAL INJURY

If you suspect a spinal injury and you cannot maintain an open airway in the position you found them, care must be taken in moving them.

Keep the casualty's back straight and support the head throughout.

It would be extremely useful to have help in moving the casualty.

The trained person should assume control when moving them.

11 If you have a bystander available to you, then this is the time to send them to call for an ambulance ensuring they have all the appropriate information, and in particular, the condition of the casualty

12 If you have no bystander, you must call for an ambulance yourself

If they have to be kept in the recovery position for **more than 30 minutes** turn them to the opposite side to relieve the pressure on the lower arm.

You must continue to monitor their breathing whilst waiting for the emergency services to take over. If they stop breathing normally, then you must call the emergency services with an update and commence CPR immediately.

It will also be worth monitoring and noting other changes such as colouration of the skin, their temperature and responsiveness levels.

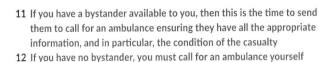

PREGNANT WOMEN

Always put an unresponsive pregnant woman in the recovery position on her **left side**. This prevents compression of the Inferior vena cava (large vein) by the uterus, which could be fatal for both the mother and the child.

Our ability to breathe is thanks to our respiratory system which is made up primarily of our airways and our lungs.

We are able to breathe in and out spontaneously providing we have air to breathe and the airways are open.

Air breathed in

- ■ Nitrogen - 78%
- □ Oxygen - 21%
- ▨ Argon and other gases - 1%

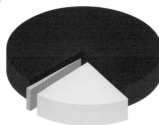

COMPOSITION OF AIR

When we breathe in the diaphragm contracts and flattens, the ribs are elevated, and as negative pressure is produced in the chest cavity, there is increased pressure in the abdomen. This draws air into the lungs to equalise the pressure.

We exhale when the diaphragm relaxes and the chest wall and lung tissue returns to their original size.

Respiration is achieved through the mouth, nose, trachea, lungs, and diaphragm. Oxygen enters the respiratory system through the mouth and the nose. The oxygen then passes through the larynx (where speech sounds are produced) and the trachea which is a tube that enters the chest cavity. In the chest cavity, the trachea splits into two smaller tubes called the bronchi. Each bronchus then divides again forming the bronchioles. These bronchial tubes lead directly into the lungs where they divide into many smaller tubes which connect to tiny sacs called alveoli. The average adult's lungs contain about 600 million of these spongy, air-filled sacs that are surrounded by capillaries. The inhaled oxygen passes into the alveoli and then enters the capillaries (diffusion) into the arterial blood which is taken back to the heart for circulating around the body.

Meanwhile, the waste-rich blood from the veins releases its carbon dioxide into the alveoli. The carbon dioxide follows the same path out of the lungs when you breathe out.

Approximately 25% of the available oxygen in each breath is used, as our body can only cope with so much each time we breathe in.

Carbon dioxide and other non-essential gases are breathed out and the whole process is repeated between 10 – 20 times per minute for an average adult.

The Respiratory System

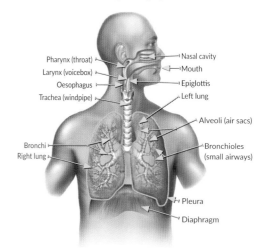

Pharynx (throat)
Larynx (voicebox)
Oesophagus
Trachea (windpipe)
Nasal cavity
Mouth
Epiglottis
Left lung
Alveoli (air sacs)
Bronchi
Right lung
Bronchioles (small airways)
Pleura
Diaphragm

Cardiopulmonary resuscitation (CPR) is an emergency procedure which is attempted in an effort to return life to a person who is not breathing normally for themselves.

This procedure combines chest compressions with rescue breaths. The chest compression replaces the heart's ability to pump oxygenated blood around the body, particularly to the vital organs such as the brain.

Rescue breathing provides the casualty, who is unable to breathe normally for themselves, valuable oxygen that is transported around the body by the chest compressions.

Without oxygen, brain damage can occur within three minutes. Therefore, your immediate action is paramount.

Referring back to Primary Survey, i.e. DR ABC, then you will have established that your casualty is not breathing normally.

Your immediate action now is to contact the emergency services and ask for an ambulance, ensuring that you state that your casualty is not breathing normally.

If you have a bystander at hand, then send them to make this important call. You can also ask your bystander to find and bring an Automated External Defibrillator (AED) to you, if one is available.

However, if you are on your own, then you must call the emergency services yourself. Stay with the casualty when making this call if possible.

If you are able to, activate the speaker function on your phone to aid communication between you and the emergency services.

Commence CPR without delay.

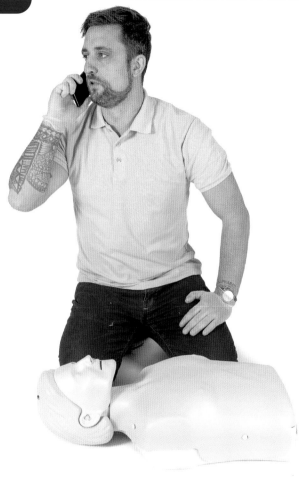

1. START WITH 30 CHEST COMPRESSIONS

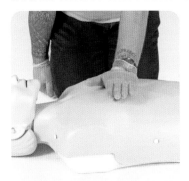

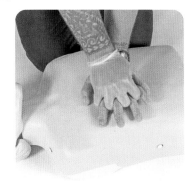

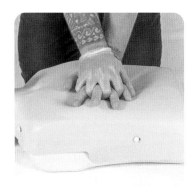

- Kneel by the side of your casualty
- Place the heel of one hand in the centre of the casualty's chest (which is the lower half of the casualty's breastbone (sternum)

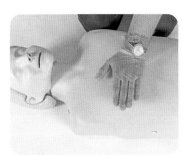

- Place the heel of your other hand on top of the first hand
- Interlock the fingers of your hands and ensure that pressure is not applied over their ribs. Do not apply any pressure over the upper abdomen or the bottom end of the sternum
- Position yourself vertically above their chest and, with your arms straight, press down on the sternum approximately 5cm
(But not more than 6cm)

- After each compression, release all the pressure on the chest without losing contact between your hands and the sternum. Do not lean on the chest.
- Repeat 30 chest compressions at a speed of 100 - 120 compressions per minute with as few interruptions as possible
- Compression and release should take an equal amount of time

In most circumstances it will be possible to identify the correct hand position for chest compressions, without removing the casualty's clothes. If you are in any doubt, then remove outer clothing.

2. GIVE 2 RESCUE BREATHS After 30 chest compressions open the airway again using head tilt and chin lift.

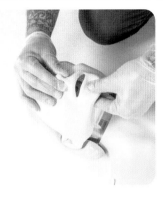

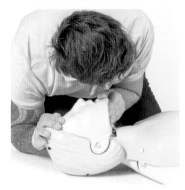

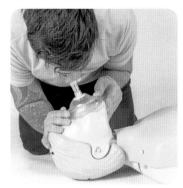

- Pinch the soft part of their nose closed, using the index finger and thumb of your hand on their forehead
- Allow their mouth to open, but maintain chin lift
- Take a normal breath and place your lips around their mouth, making sure that you have a good seal
- Blow steadily into their mouth whilst watching for their chest to rise, taking about one second as in normal breathing; this is an effective rescue breath

- Maintaining head tilt and chin lift, watch for their chest to fall as air comes out
- Take another normal breath and blow into the casualty's mouth once more to achieve a total of two effective rescue breaths. Do not interrupt compressions by more than 10 seconds to deliver two breaths. Then return your hands without delay to the correct position on the sternum and give a further 30 chest compressions

If the initial rescue breath of each sequence does not make the chest rise as in normal breathing, then, before your next attempt:

- Check the casualty's mouth and remove any visible obstruction
- Re-check that there is adequate head tilt and chin lift
- Do not attempt more than two breaths each time before returning to chest compressions

In order to reduce the risk of cross-contamination, there are various protective shields and masks available that will significantly reduce this risk. For more information about infection control please see page 11.

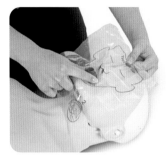 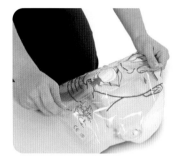 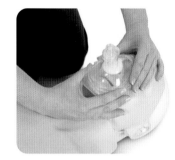

Repeat 30 compressions and 2 breaths until

- **A health professional tells you to stop**
- **The casualty is definitely waking up, moving, opening their eyes and breathing normally**
- **You become exhausted**

It is rare for CPR alone to restart the heart. Unless you are certain the casualty has recovered, continue with CPR.

Signs the casualty has recovered include:

- **Waking up**
- **Moving**
- **Opens eyes**

 AND

- **They start breathing normally again**

Be prepared to restart CPR immediately if the casualty deteriorates.

It must be emphasised that if you are unable to give rescue breaths for whatever reason, then you must continue with chest-compression-only CPR.

If there is more than one rescuer present, another should take over CPR about every 1-2 minutes to prevent fatigue.

Ensure the minimum of delay during the changeover of rescuers and do not interrupt chest compressions.

IF YOU HAVE ACCESS TO AN AED

As soon as it arrives, switch it on and attach the electrode pads on the casualty's chest. Follow the voice prompts. If more than one rescuer is present, CPR should be continued whilst the electrode pads are being attached to the chest. (See pages 26-29 for AED use).

THE CHAIN OF SURVIVAL

It is critical that you follow this chain when you are dealing with a casualty who is not breathing normally.

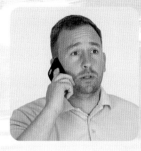 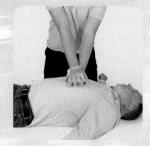 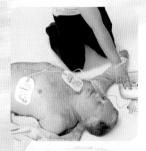 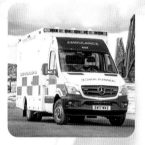

Early recognition and call for help

Recognise those at risk of cardiac arrest, and call for help in the hope that early treatment can prevent arrest.

Early CPR

Start CPR to buy time until medical help arrives.

Early defibrillation

Defibrillators give an electric shock to re-organise the rhythm of the heart.

Defibrillation within 3–5 minutes of cardiac arrest can produce survival rates as high as 50–70%.

Each minute of delay to defibrillation reduces the probability of survival to hospital discharge by 10%.

Post-resuscitation care

Provide professional help in order to restore the quality of life.

DEFIBRILLATION

When the AED arrives, you must immediately unpack it and prepare to fix the pads to the casualty. If you have trained help, then allow them to continue with CPR until you are ready. If not, then stop CPR and unpack it yourself.

If your casualty is wearing a wired bra, then this must be removed or cut through to expose the chest, particularly the area where the pads are to be fixed. Similarly, if your casualty is wearing jewellery that may come into contact with the pads, then it must be removed.

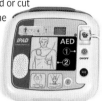

The majority of pads will be clearly marked on where they should be fixed. Depending on the make and model of the AED, the pads will generally come as two separate pads. Some will come as a single pad. Ensure that the film that is protecting the sticky pads is removed.

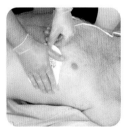

If your casualty has a pacemaker fitted, then ensure that the pads are placed at least 10cms away from it.

Do not place the pads directly on top of it. A pacemaker should be clearly identifiable, from a scar or what appears to be a small plate under the skin.

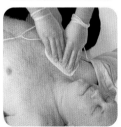

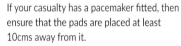

It may be necessary to prepare the casualty's chest in order for the pads to adhere. Do not waste valuable time shaving inappropriately.

Most AED pads are labelled left and right, or carry a picture of the placement. It does not matter if these pads are reversed. What is important is that should they be placed the wrong way round, they must be left in place because the adhesive may well be removed or compromised if you swap them around.

In respect of switching the AED on, they will vary from one AED to another. Some will switch themselves on as soon as the lid is removed or opened. Others will have a button to press to switch it on.

It is important that you familiarise yourself with the AED you have.

All AED's will have a voice prompt and it is important that you follow these prompts.

Some AED's will also have a screen giving you the commands.

This can be a very useful aid for those who are hard of hearing.

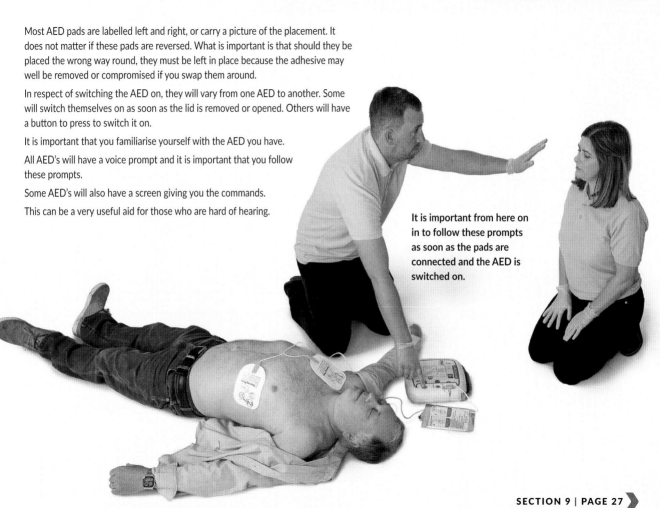

It is important from here on in to follow these prompts as soon as the pads are connected and the AED is switched on.

The AED will need to analyse the heart's rhythm. You will be prompted to ensure that no-one is touching the casualty, including yourself. Anyone touching the casualty could have an adverse effect on detecting the correct rhythm of your casualty's heart.

Dependent on the model you have, analysis will automatically

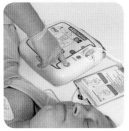

happen, or you may have to push the 'Analyse' button.

You have to take control of the situation and move people away from the casualty.

Your next prompt could be to shock the casualty. Your AED may do this automatically, or you may have to press the 'Shock' button.

Again, manage the situation and ensure that no-one is touching the casualty.

Keep following the prompts from the AED.

If you are prompted to commence CPR, then quality CPR is important.

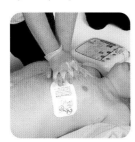

Ensure that you compress at the right depth (5-6cms) and at the right speed (100-120 chest compressions per minute).

In essence you must continue with CPR until the AED tells you to stop to either analyse the casualty's heart rhythm, or it decides that a shock should be given.

Under the current Resuscitation guidelines, you will be administering CPR for two minutes before the AED will prompt you to stop in order for it to analyse the heart's rhythm.

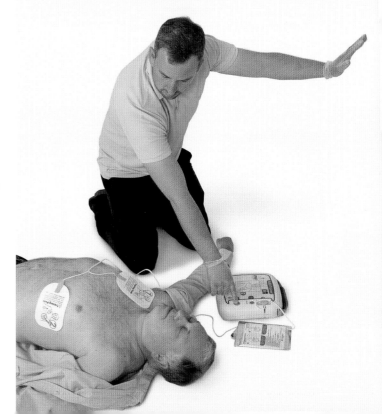

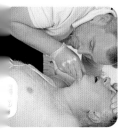
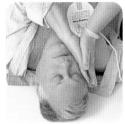
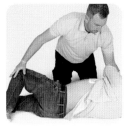
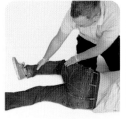
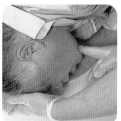
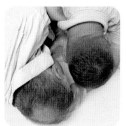

You must continue to follow the prompts until professional medical help takes over from you, your casualty recovers, or you become too exhausted to continue. Recovery will mean that your casualty shows signs of regaining responsiveness, such as coughing, opening their eyes, speaking or moving purposefully AND they start to breathe normally for themselves. To ensure they are breathing normally, conduct a breathing check.

If you are confident that they are breathing normally, place them in the recovery position with the pads attached and connected to the AED.

You must continue to monitor their breathing until professional medical help arrives and takes over from you.

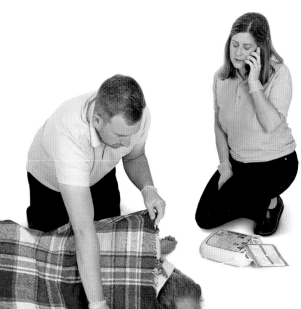

PAEDIATRIC RESUSCITATION

The term paediatric refers to children and infants (babies). A child is deemed as being aged 1 year old through to 18 years old, and an infant being aged under 1 year old.

If you are in any doubt regarding the age of the child, then treat them as an adult, as little harm will come to them by adopting the adult protocols.

As with any incident, you must carry out a primary survey.

The contents of this survey can be remembered easily by using the mnemonic **DR ABC**.

DANGERS

Make sure the area is safe

RESPONSE

Check for a response.

If they are responsive by answering or moving;

- **Leave the child in the position in which you find them** (provided they are not in further danger)
- **Check their condition and get help if needed**
- **Reassess their condition regularly**

If they are not responsive, then:

- **Shout for help**
- **Turn them on to their back**
- **Gently stimulate the child and ask loudly, 'Are you all right?'**
- **An infant can be stimulated by rubbing the soles of their feet with your finger**
- **Do not shake infants, or children with suspected cervical spine injuries**
- **Use their name when talking to them**

AIRWAY

Open their airway using the head tilt and chin lift manoeuvre:

- **Place your hand on their forehead and gently tilt their head back. Be very careful not to over extend this movement with an infant**
- **With two fingertips under the point of their chin, lift the child's chin. Use one finger for an infant.** In either case, do not push on the soft tissues under the chin as this may block the airway.

BREATHING

Look, listen and feel for normal breathing for no more than 10 seconds.

CPR for a non-breathing casualty

For CPR on an infant see Page 31

For CPR on a child see Page 32

If they are breathing normally:

- **Treat any injuries accordingly and put them in the recovery position**
- **Call for an ambulance if the injuries or condition requires it**
- **Continue to monitor their breathing**

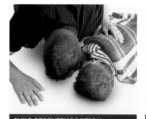

CHILD RECOVERY POSITION

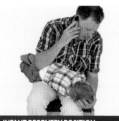

INFANT RECOVERY POSITION

CPR FOR AN INFANT

IF YOU HAVE HELP AVAILABLE ask them to call for an ambulance immediately and to bring back an AED if they can find one.

The following modifications to the adult sequence will make it more suitable for use in infants:

- Carefully remove any obvious airway obstructions
- Give 5 initial rescue breaths

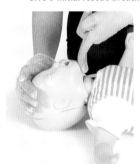

Take a breath and cover the mouth and nose of the infant with your mouth, making sure you have a good seal. If both the nose and mouth cannot be covered in the older infant, then attempt to seal only the infant's nose or mouth with your mouth (if the nose is used, close the lips to prevent air escape and vice versa).

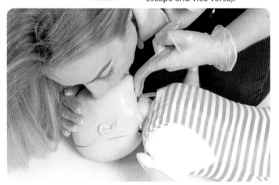

IF YOU ARE ON YOUR OWN, perform CPR for 1 minute i.e. approximately 2 cycles of 30 chest compressions followed by 2 rescue breaths.

You must then call 999 for an ambulance yourself.

TECHNIQUE FOR GIVING CHEST COMPRESSIONS FOR AN INFANT

- Compress the chest by at least one-third of its depth which is approximately 4cm for an infant
- Use the tips of 2 fingers to compress the chest
- The compression rate should be between 100–120 per minute

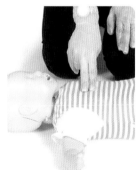

Continue with CPR (30:2) until the emergency services take over from you, your casualty recovers* or you become too exhausted to continue.

Should an AED arrive, unpack it and connect it to your casualty. Follow the voice prompts.

* Recovery means that they start to show signs of life i.e. they wake up, or start moving, or open their eyes and they start to breathe normally for themselves.

2 FINGER CHEST COMPRESSIONS

CPR FOR A CHILD

IF YOU HAVE HELP AVAILABLE ask them to call for an ambulance immediately and to bring back an AED if they can find one.

The following modifications to the adult sequence will make it more suitable for use in children:

- Carefully remove any obvious airway obstructions
- Give 5 initial rescue breaths

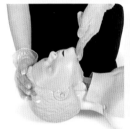 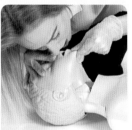

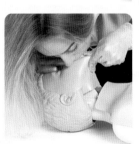

IF YOU ARE ON YOUR OWN, perform CPR for 1 minute i.e. approximately 2 cycles of 30 chest compressions followed by 2 rescue breaths.

You must then call 999 for an ambulance yourself.

TECHNIQUE FOR GIVING CHEST COMPRESSIONS FOR A CHILD

- Compress the chest by at least one-third of its depth which is approximately 5cm for a child
- Use one or two hands for a child over 1 year to achieve an adequate depth of compression
- The compression rate should be between 100–120 per minute

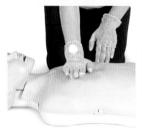 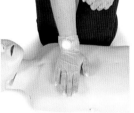

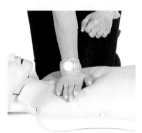

Continue with CPR (30:2) until the emergency services take over from you, your casualty recovers* or you become too exhausted to continue.

Should an AED arrive, unpack it and connect it to your casualty. Follow the voice prompts.

* Recovery means that they start to show signs of life i.e. they wake up, or start moving, or open their eyes **and** they start to breathe normally for themselves.

DROWNING

Drowning is defined as respiratory impairment from being in, or under a liquid, normally water.

Drowning begins as a result of the casualty not being able to breathe because the airways are submerged below the surface of the liquid.

As with any incident, follow the Primary Survey protocol:

D **D**ANGERS

Consider the risk to yourself before attempting to rescue the casualty.

It may well be that chemicals are involved causing an additional toxic risk e.g. a slurry tank.

R **R**ESPONSE

Check for a response as you would normally do.

A **A**IRWAY

Open the airway

B **B**REATHING

Check to see if they are breathing normally.

C **C**PR

If they are not breathing normally, shout for help and call 999 unless you have help at hand and then send them to make the call and to find an AED.

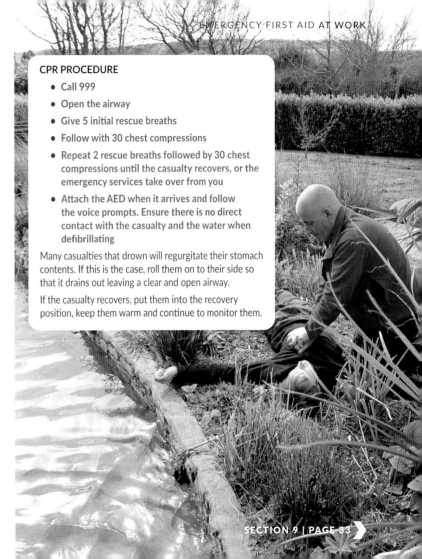

CPR PROCEDURE

- Call 999
- Open the airway
- Give 5 initial rescue breaths
- Follow with 30 chest compressions
- Repeat 2 rescue breaths followed by 30 chest compressions until the casualty recovers, or the emergency services take over from you
- Attach the AED when it arrives and follow the voice prompts. Ensure there is no direct contact with the casualty and the water when defibrillating

Many casualties that drown will regurgitate their stomach contents. If this is the case, roll them on to their side so that it drains out leaving a clear and open airway.

If the casualty recovers, put them into the recovery position, keep them warm and continue to monitor them.

There are many factors that can contribute to a respiratory disorder, including asthma, hypoxia, smoke inhalation and choking.

Choking is probably the most common of the disorders and probably the most distressing to suffer and to deal with.

Your immediate treatment is required. Should your casualty become unresponsive as a result of choking, then you will have to start resuscitation.

You should suspect choking if someone is unable to speak or talk, particularly if they're eating.

Recognition of someone choking

- Difficulty in speaking and breathing
- Coughing or gagging
- Clutching at the throat and pointing to the mouth
- Pale, grey/blue skin tone in the later stages (cyanosis)
- Ultimately – unresponsiveness

If your casualty shows signs of a mild or partial airway obstruction then:

- Encourage them to cough
- Stay calm and offer plenty of encouragement and reassurance

If coughing becomes ineffective then provide treatment for a severe airway obstruction for an adult:

- Check their mouth and remove any obvious obstruction

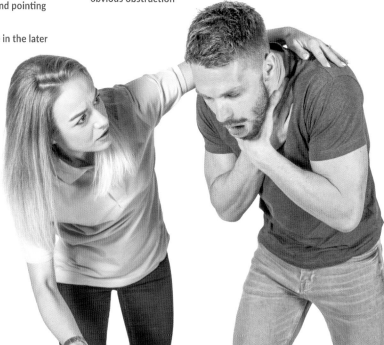

Bend them forward and give up to five back blows

- Stand to the side and slightly behind your casualty

- Support the chest with one hand and lean them forward so that when the obstructing object is dislodged it comes out of the mouth rather than to go further down the airway

- Give up to five sharp blows between their shoulder blades with the heel of your other hand

Check to see if each back blow has relieved the airway obstruction. The aim is to relieve the obstruction with each blow rather than to give all five unnecessarily.

Continued on page 36.

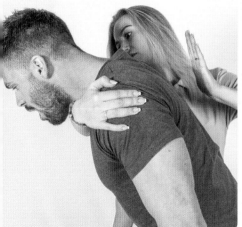

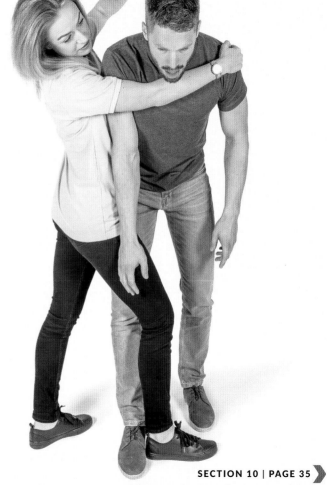

Give them up to five abdominal thrusts

- Stand behind your casualty and put both arms round the upper part of their abdomen

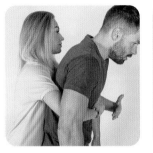 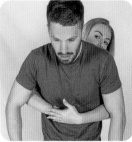 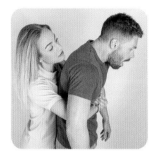 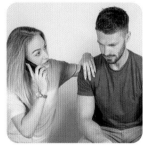

- Lean them forward
- Clench your fist and place it between the umbilicus (navel) and the bottom end of their sternum (breastbone)

- Grasp this hand with your other hand and pull sharply inwards and upwards
- Repeat up to five times

- Check to see if each abdominal thrust has relieved the airway obstruction. The aim is to relieve the obstruction with each thrust rather than to give all five unnecessarily

- If you have performed abdominal thrusts on a casualty, they must be sent to hospital to be examined for any internal injuries.

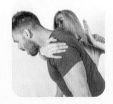

If the obstruction cannot be removed after the first cycle of back blows and abdominal thrusts, then you must call for an ambulance immediately.

Repeat the process of up to five back blows followed by up to five abdominal thrusts until the casualty recovers, or the emergency medical services take over from you.

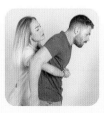

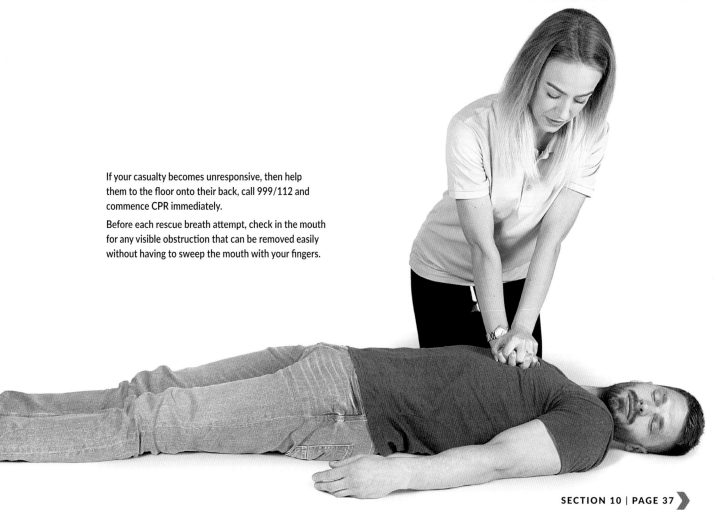

If your casualty becomes unresponsive, then help them to the floor onto their back, call 999/112 and commence CPR immediately.

Before each rescue breath attempt, check in the mouth for any visible obstruction that can be removed easily without having to sweep the mouth with your fingers.

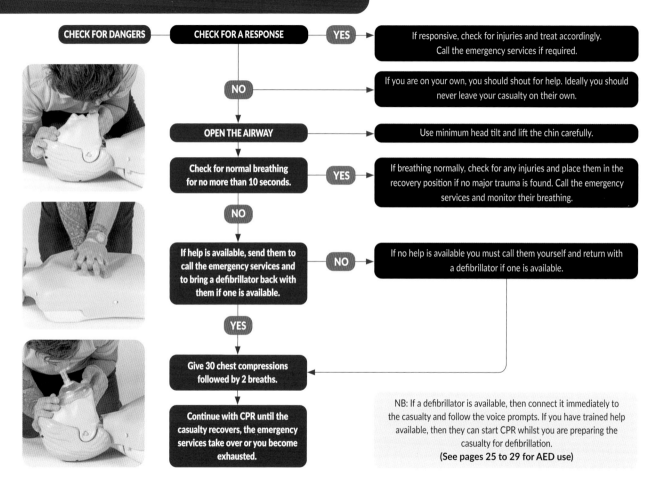

CHECK FOR DANGERS → **CHECK FOR A RESPONSE** → **YES** → If responsive, check for injuries and treat accordingly. Call the emergency services if required.

NO → If you are on your own, you should shout for help. Ideally you should never leave your casualty on their own.

OPEN THE AIRWAY → Use minimum head tilt and lift the chin carefully.

Check for normal breathing for no more than 10 seconds. → **YES** → If breathing normally, check for any injuries and place them in the recovery position if no major trauma is found. Call the emergency services and monitor their breathing.

NO

If help is available, send them to call the emergency services and to bring a defibrillator back with them if one is available. → **NO** → If no help is available you must call them yourself and return with a defibrillator if one is available.

YES

Give 30 chest compressions followed by 2 breaths.

Continue with CPR until the casualty recovers, the emergency services take over or you become exhausted.

NB: If a defibrillator is available, then connect it immediately to the casualty and follow the voice prompts. If you have trained help available, then they can start CPR whilst you are preparing the casualty for defibrillation.
(See pages 25 to 29 for AED use)

The circulatory system is our body's transport system for two fluids, namely, blood and lymph.

For the purposes of first aid we will focus on the transport of blood, also known as the cardiovascular system.

This system consists of the heart and blood vessels, which supply our body, and in particular, our vital organs such as the brain and heart, with blood containing oxygen and nutrients to keep them healthy.

Our heart is a hollow muscular pump, about the size of your fist, with two pairs of chambers. These chambers collect blood flowing back from our body after depositing the oxygen and nutrients, before being pumped back to the lungs to collect more oxygen so that the cycle of transportation can continue.

The adult heart beats approximately 60 – 80 times every minute and pumps approximately six litres of blood around our body every minute.

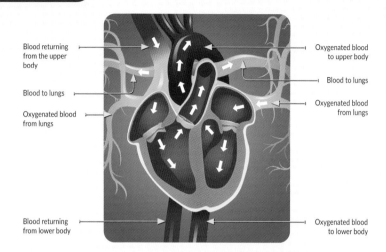

Blood returning from the upper body

Blood to lungs

Oxygenated blood from lungs

Blood returning from lower body

Oxygenated blood to upper body

Blood to lungs

Oxygenated blood from lungs

Oxygenated blood to lower body

The blood vessels within this system are:

- **Arteries**
  Deliver oxygenated blood from the heart to the body, with the exception of the pulmonary artery which carries de-oxygenated blood from the heart to the lungs

- **Veins**
  Carry the de-oxygenated blood back to the heart

- **Capillaries**
  Much smaller vessels that form a link between the arteries, veins and body tissue to allow the transfer of oxygen and nutrients to the body and the waste products to be removed

Blood is made up of:

- **Plasma**
  The fluid component of the blood of which 90% is water

- **Platelets**
  Help to block the blood flow by clotting

- **Red cells**
  Transport the oxygen via the haemoglobin

- **White cells**
  Manufacture antibodies and fight infection and bacteria

HYPOVOLAEMIC SHOCK

There are a number of reasons why this system could fail, including blood loss, failure of the heart, poor circulation, a fall in blood pressure and the lack of oxygen contained within the body.

Other conditions include poisoning, vomiting, infection, burns and injury to the spinal cord, but this is by no means the definitive list.

As a First Aider, there are a number of things we can do for our casualty such as to stop the bleeding and to take pressure off the heart. This will be covered later, but one of your main concerns should be that shock will set in very quickly if you don't react quickly enough, and shock can be a killer!

Hypovolaemic shock is best described as a failure or collapse of the circulatory system when the arterial blood pressure is too low to provide an adequate blood supply to the tissues.

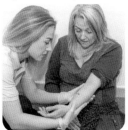 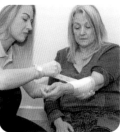

Signs and symptoms of hypovolaemic shock

- **Ashen coloured skin** (grey/blue)
- **Clammy and cold skin to touch**
- **Feeling of sickness and thirst**
- **Their breathing will be rapid and shallow**
- **Rapid, weak pulse**

Treatment of hypovolaemic shock

- Deal with the injury or condition
- Make them comfortable and lay them down
- Raise both legs providing it does not compromise their injuries further
- Keep them warm and maintain their response levels by talking to them
- Call for an ambulance
- Monitor their response and breathing
- Do not allow them to smoke, eat or drink as it may affect their well-being and it could compromise further treatment

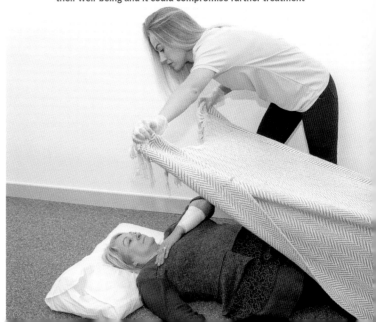

FAINTING

Fainting is a sudden, usually temporary, brief loss of responsiveness generally caused by insufficient oxygen in the brain.

The signs and symptoms are the same as shock with the exception that the pulse rate is slower.

A casualty who has fainted will generally make a rapid recovery and feel fine very quickly.

TREATMENT FOR SOMEONE WHO FEELS FAINT

- Help them to the floor and lie them down
- Raise and support their legs
- Offer them plenty of fresh air
- Sit them up gradually
- Comfort and reassure them

TREATMENT FOR SOMEONE WHO HAS FAINTED

If a person faints and does not regain responsiveness within one or two minutes, you should put them into the recovery position, monitor their breathing, and medical assistance should be sought.

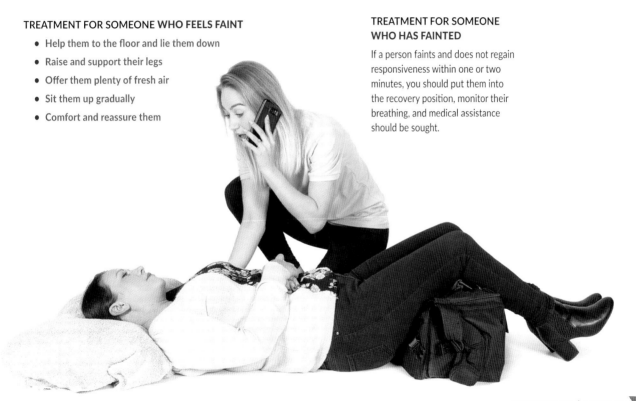

A wound can be best described as a type of injury in which the skin is torn, cut or punctured (an open wound), or where a blunt force created a contusion (a bruise).

In first aid there are 6 types of wounds that you should be familiar with:

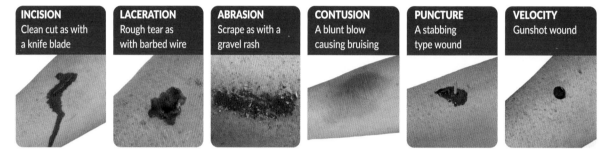

INCISION
Clean cut as with a knife blade

LACERATION
Rough tear as with barbed wire

ABRASION
Scrape as with a gravel rash

CONTUSION
A blunt blow causing bruising

PUNCTURE
A stabbing type wound

VELOCITY
Gunshot wound

When a blood vessel is torn or severed, blood loss and shock cause the blood pressure to fall and the injured vessels will contract at the site of injury.

Platelets and proteins come into contact with the injured site and plug the wound.

This clotting process begins within ten minutes if the loss of blood is brought under control.

BLEEDING IS CLASSIFIED BY THE TYPE OF BLOOD VESSEL THAT IS DAMAGED.

Arterial Pumps from the wound with the heartbeat

Venous Gushes from the wound or pools at the site

Capillary Oozing at the site of injury

Once you have completed your initial casualty assessment for prioritising your treatment, you must follow the guidelines for personal protection and hygiene control before you begin to treat the casualty.

Treatment for the control of bleeding

- Put on disposable gloves
- Expose and examine the wound
- Apply direct pressure with your fingers or palm, preferably over a sterile dressing or non-fluffy clean pad (you can ask your casualty to apply this pressure)
- Elevate and support the injured part for wounds that are not catastrophic
- Help the casualty to lie down and raise the legs if you suspect shock
- Secure the dressing with a bandage large enough to cover the wound
- If blood seeps through this dressing, remove both the dressing and bandage and apply pressure to the bleed with a new dressing. Apply another bandage once the bleeding is under control
- Support the injured limb with a sling or bandaging if appropriate, providing the casualty allows you to do so
- Monitor their response levels and call for an ambulance

CATASTROPHIC BLEEDING

If you are unable to stop the bleeding because of the severity, then you will need to apply direct pressure continually and then pack the wound with haemostatic dressings, or apply a tourniquet.

If you have neither, then you must continue to apply direct pressure and consider making an improvised tourniquet. It is imperative that you call for an ambulance immediately for a severe, or catastrophic bleed.

To summarise the treatment for catastrophic bleeding

- Do apply direct pressure to the wound
- Do use a haemostatic dressing or tourniquet
- Do not apply indirect pressure to proximal pressure points
- Do not elevate an extremity

Fortunately, the vast majority of businesses would never have to deal with a catastrophic bleed in a first aid situation at work. For most First Aiders, blood loss can be controlled by following the guidelines as detailed in the left hand column.

> It must be emphasised that further training is required for First Aiders in respect of using haemostatic dressings or tourniquets. Please speak to your training provider.

EMBEDDED OBJECTS

If during your examination of the wound you see an embedded object such as a piece of glass, then you must leave it in place and dress around it.

Your aim is to stop the bleeding, but care must be taken not to put any direct pressure on the embedded object.

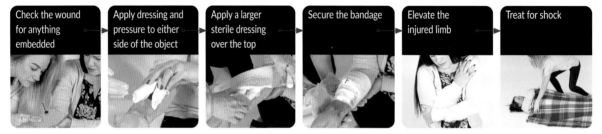

| Check the wound for anything embedded | Apply dressing and pressure to either side of the object | Apply a larger sterile dressing over the top | Secure the bandage | Elevate the injured limb | Treat for shock |

BLEEDING FROM ORIFICES

Signs, symptoms and causes

Site	Appearance	Cause
Mouth	Bright red, frothy, coughed up.	Bleeding in the lungs.
	Vomited blood, red or dark reddish brown.	Bleeding in the stomach.
Ear	Fresh bright-red blood.	Injury to ear, perforated eardrum.
	Thin, watery blood.	Head injury.
Nose	Fresh bright red blood.	Ruptured blood vessel in nostril.
	Thin, watery blood.	Skull fracture.
Anus	Fresh bright-red blood.	Injury to anus or lower bowel.
	Black tarry, offensive smelling stool.	Injury to upper bowel.
Urethra	Urine with red or smoky appearance and occasional clots.	Bleeding from the bladder, kidneys.
Vagina	Either fresh or dark blood	Menstruation, miscarriage, disease or injury to the vagina or womb.

TREATMENT

- Treat the cause where possible using sterile dressings
- Treat the casualty for shock
- Monitor their condition, particularly their breathing
- Call 999/112 for an ambulance
- Lay them injured side down where possible
- Do not try to plug the wound, but cover it with a sterile dressing
- Offer them plenty of reassurance
- Pay attention to the casualty's modesty and dignity, particularly if they are bleeding from the anus or vagina

AMPUTATIONS

Any part of the body that has been severed will need immediate hospital treatment.

There is almost certain to be severe blood loss, and your aim as an Emergency First Aider is to control the bleeding, treat for shock and to protect and transport the amputated body part to hospital with the casualty.

Your prompt and effective treatment may just allow the amputated part to be stitched back successfully with micro-surgery.

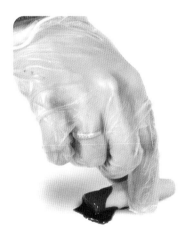
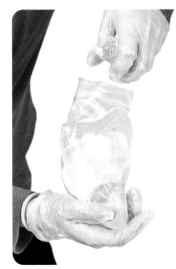

Signs and symptoms

- Bleeding
- Shock
- Severe pain in the majority of cases
- An open wound
- Amputated body part

Treatment

- Ensure that the area is safe. Turn off machinery etc, that may have caused the accident
- Control the loss of blood by applying direct pressure with a sterile, non-fluffy dressing
- Treat the casualty for shock
- Reduce the risk of cross-infection by wearing gloves
- Call 999/112 for an ambulance
- Wrap the amputated part in plastic such as cling-film
- Wrap it further in a cloth
- Submerge the wrapped and protected part in ice. It is important that the severed part does not make direct contact with the ice. Mark the package clearly with the casualty's name and ensure that it is transported to hospital with the casualty
- Protect and maintain an open airway
- Monitor their breathing. Be prepared to resuscitate the casualty if they stop breathing normally

MINOR CUTS AND GRAZES

Cuts and grazes are some of the most common injuries.

Minor cuts and grazes (where only the surface layer of skin is cut or scraped off) may bleed and feel slightly painful, but the affected area will normally scab over and heal quickly.

However, if the cut is in an area that is constantly moving, such as your knee joint, it may take longer to heal.

Depending on how deep the cut is and where it is on your body, a scar may remain once the cut has healed.

Deeper cuts may damage important structures below the skin such as nerves, blood vessels or tendons.

However, grazes that remove the deeper layers of skin are rare.

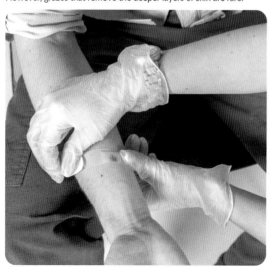

Most cuts and grazes can be easily treated by cleaning them thoroughly and covering them with a plaster or dressing.

Please bear in mind that hypoallergenic plasters are available should your casualty have an allergy to ordinary plasters.

SEEK MEDICAL HELP IF ANY OF THE BELOW APPLY:

You think there is damage to deeper tissues: signs include numbness (indicating injury to a nerve), blood spurting from the wound or bleeding that does not stop after five minutes of continuous firm pressure.

The wound is at risk of becoming infected: for example, a cut has been contaminated with soil, faeces or a dirty blade, or fragments of material such as grit or glass which can be seen in the wound.

The wound has become infected: signs include swelling of the affected area, pus coming from the wound, redness spreading from the wound and increasing pain. The wound cannot be closed with a plaster, or it starts to open up when it moves.

The wound will create an unwelcome scar: for example, if it occurs on a prominent part of the casualty's face.

TETANUS IMMUNISATION

If the wound has been contaminated by dirt or soil, then it is advisable to ask the casualty about their history of tetanus immunisation.

Advise to seek medical advice if:

- They have never been immunised
- If they are unsure about their history of injections

BRUISING

Bruises are bluish or purple-coloured patches that appear on the skin when tiny blood vessels (capillaries) break or burst underneath it.

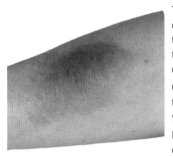

The blood from the capillaries leak into the soft tissue under the skin causing the discolouration.

Over time this fades through shades of yellow or green.

Bruises often feel tender or swollen at first.

What causes bruising?

Bruising is caused by internal bleeding (under the skin) due to a person injuring themselves by, for example, falling over, walking into something or playing sports.

Some people are naturally more likely to bruise than others, for example, the elderly may bruise more easily because their skin is thinner and the tissue underneath is more fragile.

Treatment for bruises

Treat bruises, initially, by limiting the bleeding. You can do this by cooling the area with a cold compress (a flannel or cloth soaked in cold water) or an ice pack wrapped in a towel.

To make an ice pack, place ice cubes or a packet of frozen vegetables in a plastic bag and wrap them in a towel. Hold this over the affected area for at least 10 minutes.

Do not put the ice pack straight onto the skin as this will possibly cause further damage.

Most bruises will disappear after around two weeks.

If the bruise is still there after two weeks, you should recommend that your casualty see their GP.

Internal bruising

Bruises don't just happen under the skin - they can also happen deeper in the body's tissues, organs and bones.

While the bleeding isn't visible, the bruises can cause swelling and pain.

You should recommend that your casualty seeks medical attention, or call for an ambulance if you feel the injury is of a serious nature, particularly if they have been involved in an accident.

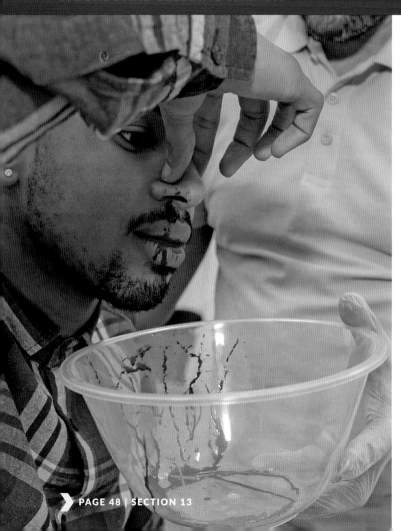

NOSEBLEEDS

A common injury that is caused generally by a direct blow or sneezing. However, high blood pressure can also cause a sudden bleed with little warning.

If the blood is watery, then it could suggest a head injury, therefore making the incident far more serious i.e. possible skull fracture.

Treatment

- Sit the casualty down and lean them forward
- Ask them to pinch the soft part of the nose as they lean forward
- Apply this pressure for 10 minutes and then release slowly
- Ask them to avoid rubbing or blowing their nose
- If you are unable to stop the bleeding, ask them to repeat the pinching process for a further 10 minutes
- If the bleeding continues beyond 30 minutes then you will need to seek medical advice

  If you suspect a head injury, then an ambulance must be summoned.

If the casualty is feeling faint or nausea you may consider sitting the casualty on the floor with their back supported. This could potentially prevent a fall.

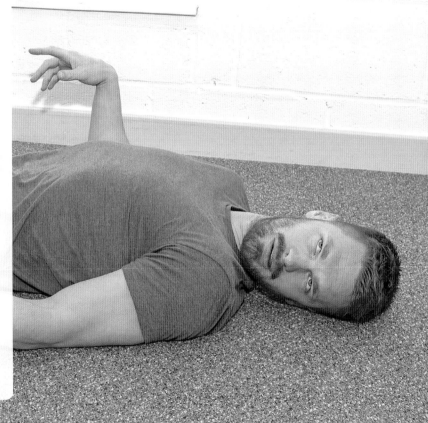

WHAT IS EPILEPSY?

Epilepsy is a condition that affects the brain. When someone has epilepsy, it means they have a tendency to have epileptic seizures.

Anyone can have a one-off seizure, but this doesn't always mean they have epilepsy. Epilepsy is usually only diagnosed if someone has had more than one seizure, and doctors think it is likely they could have more.

Epilepsy can start at any age and there are many different types. Some types of epilepsy last for a limited time and the person eventually stops having seizures. But for many people epilepsy is a life-long condition.

WHAT ARE EPILEPTIC SEIZURES?

A seizure happens when there is a sudden burst of intense electrical activity in the brain. This causes a temporary disruption to the way the brain normally works.

The result is an epileptic seizure.

There are many different types of seizure. What happens to someone during a seizure depends on which part of their brain is affected. During some types of seizure, the person may remain alert and aware of what's going on around them, and with other types they may lose awareness. They may have unusual sensations, feelings, or movements, or they may go stiff, fall to the floor and jerk.

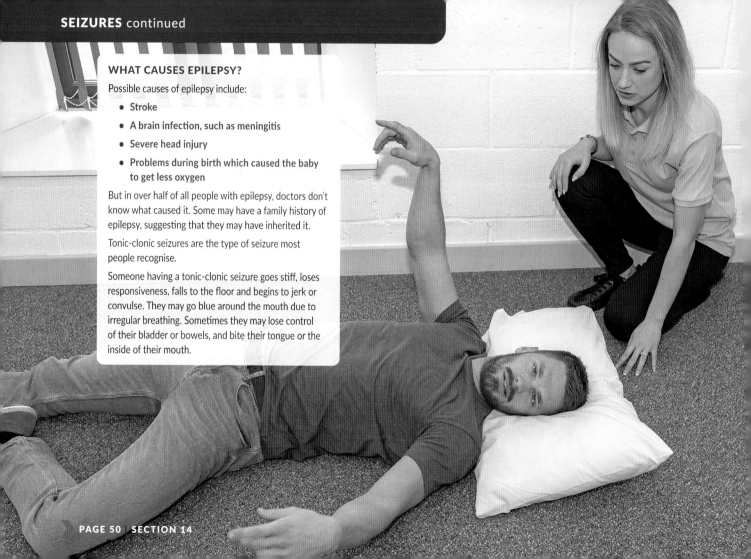

WHAT CAUSES EPILEPSY?

Possible causes of epilepsy include:

- **Stroke**
- **A brain infection, such as meningitis**
- **Severe head injury**
- **Problems during birth which caused the baby to get less oxygen**

But in over half of all people with epilepsy, doctors don't know what caused it. Some may have a family history of epilepsy, suggesting that they may have inherited it.

Tonic-clonic seizures are the type of seizure most people recognise.

Someone having a tonic-clonic seizure goes stiff, loses responsiveness, falls to the floor and begins to jerk or convulse. They may go blue around the mouth due to irregular breathing. Sometimes they may lose control of their bladder or bowels, and bite their tongue or the inside of their mouth.

HOW TO HELP IF YOU SEE SOMEONE HAVING A TONIC-CLONIC SEIZURE

Do:

- **Protect them from injury** (remove harmful objects from nearby)
- **Cushion their head**
- **Look for an epilepsy identity card or identity jewellery – it may give you information about their seizures and what to do**
- **Time how long the jerking lasts**
- **Aid breathing by gently placing them in the recovery position once the jerking has stopped**
- **Stay with the them until they are fully recovered**
- **Be calmly reassuring**

Don't:

- **Restrain their movements**
- **Put anything in their mouth**
- **Try to move them unless they are in danger**
- **Give them anything to eat or drink until they are fully recovered**
- **Attempt to bring them round**

Call for an ambulance if:

- **You know it is their first seizure**

  or

- **The jerking continues for more than five minutes**

  or

- **They have one tonic-clonic seizure after another without regaining responsiveness between seizures**

  or

- **They are injured during the seizure**

  or

- **You believe they need urgent medical attention**

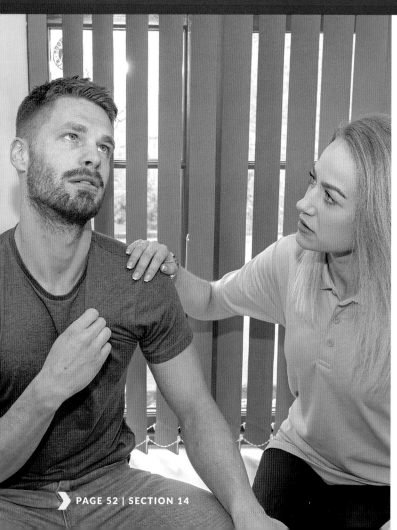

FOCAL SEIZURES

This type of seizure can also be called a partial seizure. Someone having a focal seizure may not be aware of their surroundings or what they are doing. They may have unusual movements and behaviour such as plucking at their clothes, smacking their lips, swallowing repeatedly or wandering around.

How to help if you see someone having a focal seizure.

Do:

- **Guide them away from danger** (such as roads or open water)
- **Stay with them until recovery is complete**
- **Be calmly reassuring**
- **Explain anything that they may have missed**

Don't:

- **Restrain them**
- **Act in a way that could frighten them, such as making abrupt movements or shouting at them**
- **Assume they are aware of what is happening, or what has happened**
- **Give them anything to eat or drink until they are fully recovered**
- **Attempt to bring them round**

Call for an ambulance if:

- **You know it is their first seizure**
  or
- **The seizure continues for more than five minutes**
  or
- **They are injured during the seizure**
  or
- **You believe they need urgent medical attention**

Burns and scalds are among the most serious and painful of injuries. They can be caused by a number of factors including fire, water, electricity, oils, hot surfaces, steam, chemicals and radiation.

CLASSIFICATION OF BURNS

Superficial

The outer layer of skin is burnt causing redness, tenderness and inflammation.

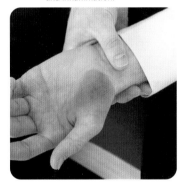

Typical factors causing this would be sunburn or touching a hot iron.

The skin is not broken or blistered.

Partial thickness

The outer layer of the skin is burnt and broken causing blistering, swelling, pain and rawness.

Full thickness

All the layers of skin have been damaged causing the skin to look pale, charred and waxy with fatty deposits. There may also be damage to the nerves.

When to send a casualty to hospital

Every year in the UK, around 175,000 people attend hospital accident and emergency departments for burns injuries.

People who may be at greater risk from the effects of burns, such as children under five years of age and pregnant women, should seek medical attention after a burn or scald.

Assessing the extent of the burn

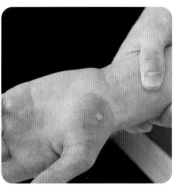

One quick way to estimate the surface area that has been burned is to compare it to the size of the palm of the casualty's hand, which is roughly equal to 1% of the body's total surface area.

For other groups, you must send them to hospital if:

- The burns affect the hands, feet, face and genital areas
- Full thickness burns
- Burns that extend around a limb
- All partial thickness burns larger than 1% of the body's surface. The casualty's hand represents about 1% on the body's surface
- All superficial burns that represent 5% of the body's surface
- Burns with a mixed pattern of depth

If you are in any doubt, then you should seek medical advice.

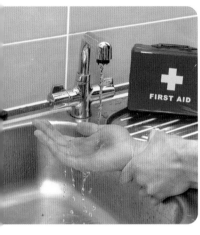

Treatment of burns

- Ensure the area is safe, particularly from the source that created the burn or scald
- Wear disposable gloves
- If it's possible, remove the watch and any jewellery around the affected area
- Cool the burn with cool running tap water for 20 minutes
- Cover the burn with a suitable sterile dressing that is not fluffy. You can cover it with cling film if you have no appropriate dressing
- Treat the casualty for shock
- Monitor their condition throughout and call for an ambulance if it deteriorates
- Remove them to hospital if you consider it appropriate

You must not:

- Apply any form of cream, ointment or fat to the affected area
- Burst any blister that may form
- Apply any form of adhesive dressing
- Remove anything that is stuck to the affected area

NB: The biggest risk associated with bursting blisters is infection

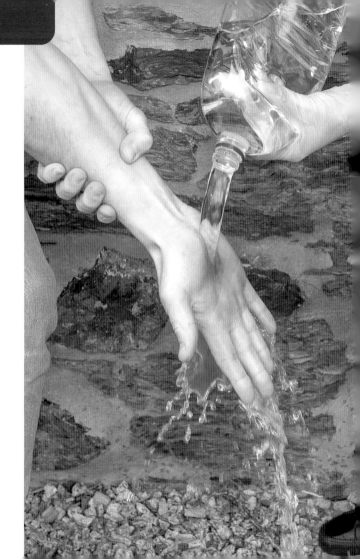

SPLINTERS

A foreign object in first aid terms, relates to an object of any size that enters the body through many of its orifices, or penetrates the skin and is embedded.

You should decide on whether you can remove it without having to seek medical help.

If a common embedded object such as a splinter is partly exposed, then it is acceptable to remove it with tweezers.

First aid tweezers generally come in a sterile package.

Washing grit away under running water can also be a useful treatment.

If this won't remove the object, then the wound should be dressed with a sterile dressing, without putting direct pressure on the object and then seek medical attention.

However, for other objects such as glass or a fishing hook, they must be left in place and you should not attempt to remove it.

Dress the wound appropriately and seek medical advice.

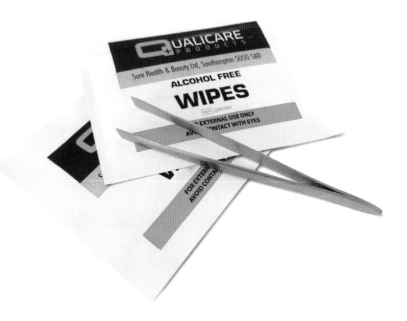

THE NOSE

- Objects pushed up the nose may cause blockages or infection. Keep your casualty calm and reassure them.
- Get the casualty to breathe through their mouth
- Do not attempt to remove the object
- Send the casualty to hospital

THE EARS

If a foreign object enters the ear and becomes lodged, it can cause damage to the ear canal, the eardrum and in some cases, cause temporary deafness.

The object should be left in the ear, unless it's a living object such as an insect that could be removed by flooding the ear with tepid water.

If this doesn't work, then you must seek medical advice.

If you need to seek medical advice:

- Cover the ear with a sterile dressing, taking care not to put any direct pressure on the object
- Send the casualty to hospital

SWALLOWED OBJECTS

Children commonly swallow small objects.

Many will enter the digestive system without choking the casualty, and leave the body in its natural way.

However, you should seek medical attention irrespective.

If you know that the object was sharp or toxic, then you must seek urgent medical attention.

If the object becomes stuck in the respiratory tract, then you should follow the choking procedure.

Some sharp objects may stick in the throat, such as fish bones or glass. If this is the case, then you must seek urgent medical attention as the airway could swell which would affect the casualty's ability to breathe normally.

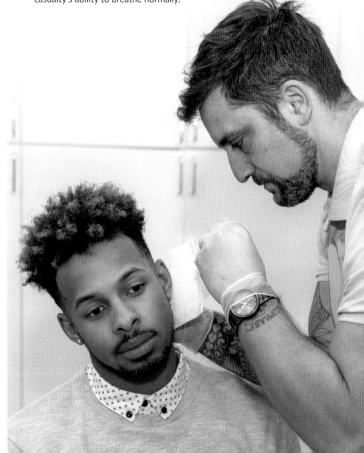